Contents

Introduction and Aims

What we eat and drink has a vital effect on our feelings of wellbeing and health. Knowledge of which foods are 'healthier' and how to cope with various special diets can have a profound effect not only on our health, but also that of our family and those we care for.

Aims

This book has been designed to provide general information on nutrition and health. Nutrition is simply the study of the function of nutrients (the components which are found in foods and drinks) and their effect on the body.

It aims to give anyone with an interest in nutrition an insight into the subject so that they can make more informed choices about their own diet and that of others.

The book also aims to give the reader some time for reflection and consideration at the end of each section.

The book has also been compiled for students to accompany the Level 1 and Level 2 Awards in Healthier Food and Special Diets from the Royal Society for Public Health. These qualifications are ideal for anyone involved in:

- Catering and cooking
- Caring in hospitals or residential care
- The hospitality and leisure industry
- Food production
- Retail
- Education
- Health and nutrition support

The Royal Society for Public Health is an independent, multi-disciplinary organisation, dedicated to the promotion and protection of collective human health and wellbeing. It provides various accredited qualifications in healthier foods and special diets, nutrition and other related health topics like food safety and health improvement.

This book aims to introduce various topics on food and nutrition including:

- Government bodies and key organisations involved in food and nutrition
- Sources of nutrients from foods and fluids
- Diet and health which looks at the way food can impact on our health
- Special diets including obesity, coeliac disease, diabetes, raised cholesterol levels and allergies
- Nutrition at various life stages from birth to old age

- Good catering practices including cooking and food labelling, as well as sources of information
- A summary and list of resources which gives ideas for other sources of information and encourages the reader to take studies further.

Reader Reflections

Think about why you are reading this book. Think of three key things you want to know about healthier foods and special diets.

Do you know anyone who has any health problems that may be related to a poor diet?

Government Bodies and Key Organisations

A healthy diet has a profound effect on the health of populations. Also, various types of health problems can be a major cost to the economy as treatments and support are provided to those with health problems.

Conditions Related to an Unhealthy Diet

Various conditions are thought to have a dietary component in their development. These include:

- Obesity
- Dental decay (caries)
- High blood pressure and strokes
- Type II diabetes
- Constipation and other bowel problems
- Cancers of various types
- Coronary Heart Disease (CHD)
- Liver disease
- Rickets and other bone health problems
- Anaemia of various types
- Malnutrition and being underweight
- Liver disease

The Government has various strategies to help with these. Some of these are aimed at providing information and advice to individuals and others set policies for organisations dealing with specific groups of the population.

'Healthy Lives, Healthy People'

This is the HM Government White Paper on Public Health, published in 2010, which discusses the Government strategy for health. It seeks to reduce the alarming levels of lifestyle driven health problems such as obesity.

Department of Health

The Department of Health provides strategic leadership for public health, the NHS and social care in England. The Department of Health's purpose is to improve England's health and wellbeing and in doing so achieve better health, better care, and better value for all. It produces extensive information on diet and health.

The Department of Health provides information on all aspects of health on its website.

The eatwell plate

Use the eatwell plate to help you get the balance right. It shows how much of what you eat should come from each food group.

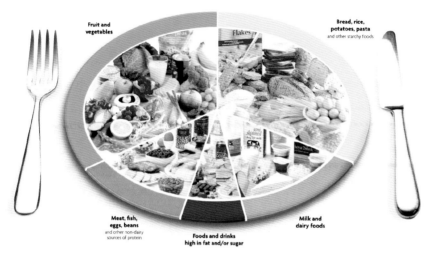

Fruit and vegetables

Bread, rice, potatoes, pasta and other starchy foods

Meat, fish, eggs, beans and other non-dairy sources of protein

Foods and drinks high in fat and/or sugar

Milk and dairy foods

Department of Health in association with the Welsh Assembly Government, the Scottish Government and the Food Standards Agency in Northern Ireland

One of its key websites is NHS Choices (see Resources list), which gives good information on a healthy nutritious diet and tips to help achieve this.

It also includes the well known eatwell plate which shows how much of what you eat should come from each food group.

Eight Tips for Eating Well are Used to Give a Good Basis for a Healthy Diet

1. Base your meals on starchy foods

Starchy foods include potatoes, cereals, pasta, rice and bread. Choose wholegrain varieties when you can; they contain more fibre and can make you feel full for longer. Starchy foods should make up around one third of the foods you eat. Most of us should . eat more starchy foods. Try to include at least one starchy food with each main meal. Some people think starchy foods are fattening, but gram for gram they contain fewer than half the calories of fat.

2. Eat lots of fruit and vegetables

It is recommended that we eat at least five portions of different types of fruit and vegetables a day. This is easier than it sounds. A glass of 100% unsweetened fruit juice can count as one portion and vegetables cooked into dishes also count. Why not chop a banana over your breakfast cereal or swap your usual mid-morning snack for some dried fruit?

3. Eat more fish

Fish is a good source of protein and contains many vitamins and minerals. Aim for at least two portions a week, including at least one portion of oily fish. Oily fish is high in omega-3 fats, which may help to prevent heart disease. You can choose from fresh, frozen and canned; but remember that canned and smoked fish can be high in salt. Oily fish include salmon, mackerel, trout, herring, fresh tuna, sardines and pilchards. Non-oily fish include haddock, plaice, coley, cod, tinned tuna, skate and hake. Anyone who regularly eats a lot of fish should try to choose as wide a variety as possible.

4. Cut down on saturated fat and sugar

We all need some fat in our diet. But it's important to pay attention to the amount and type of fat we're eating. There are two main types of fat: saturated and unsaturated. Too much saturated fat can increase the amount of cholesterol in the blood, which increases your risk of developing heart disease. Saturated fat is found in many foods, such as hard cheese, cakes, biscuits, sausages, cream, butter, lard and pies. Try to cut down and choose foods that contain unsaturated rather than saturated fats, such as vegetable oils, oily fish and avocados. For a healthier choice, use just a small amount of vegetable oil or reduced fat spread instead of butter, lard or ghee. When you're having meat, choose lean cuts and cut off any visible fat.

Most people in the UK eat and drink too much sugar. Sugary foods and drinks, including alcoholic drinks, are often high in calories, and could contribute to weight gain. They can also cause tooth decay, especially if eaten between meals. Cut down on sugary fizzy drinks, alcoholic drinks, cakes, biscuits and pastries, which contain added sugars. Added sugar is the kind of sugar we should be cutting down on rather than sugars that are found naturally in foods such as fruit and milk. Food labels can help; use them to check how much sugar foods contain. More than 15g of sugar per 100g means that the food is high in sugar.

5. Eat less salt

Even if you don't add salt to your food, you may still be eating too much. About three-quarters of the salt we eat is already in the food we buy, such as breakfast cereals, soups, breads and sauces. Eating too much salt can raise your blood pressure and people with high blood pressure are more likely to develop heart disease or have a stroke. Use food labels to help you cut down. More than 1.5g of salt per 100g means the food is high in salt. Adults and children over 11 should eat no more than 6g of salt a day. Younger children should have even less.

6. Get active and be a healthy weight

Eating a healthy, balanced diet plays an important part in maintaining a healthy weight, which is an important part of overall good health. Being overweight or obese can lead to health conditions such as type 2 diabetes, certain cancers, heart disease and stroke. Being underweight could also affect your health. Most adults need to lose weight and need to eat fewer calories in order to do this.

If you're trying to lose weight, aim to eat less and be more active. Eating a healthy, balanced diet will help. Aim to cut down on foods that are high in fat and sugar, and eat plenty of fruit and vegetables. Don't forget that alcohol is also high in calories, so cutting down can help you to control your weight. If you're worried about your weight, ask your GP or a dietitian for advice. Physical activity can help you to maintain weight loss or be a healthy weight. Being active doesn't have to mean hours at the gym; you can find ways to fit more activity into your daily life.

7. Don't get thirsty

We need to drink about 1.5 litres of fluid (6-8 cups or glasses) every day to stop us getting dehydrated. This is in addition to the fluid we get from the food we eat. All non-alcoholic drinks count, but water, milk and fruit juices are the healthiest. Try to avoid sugary, soft and fizzy drinks that are high in added sugars and can be high in calories and bad for teeth. When the weather is warm or when we get active, we may need more.

8. Don't skip breakfast

Some people skip breakfast because they think it will help them lose weight. In fact, research shows that eating breakfast can help people control their weight. A healthy breakfast is an important part of a balanced diet, and provides some of the vitamins and minerals we need for good health. Wholemeal cereal with fruit sliced over the top is a tasty and nutritious breakfast.

Food Standards Agency

The Food Standards Agency is an independent government department set up by an Act of Parliament in 2000 to protect the public's health and consumer interests in relation to food. This includes information on food allergies. It used to deal with nutrition as well as food safety.

Children's Food Trust

Established in 2005, the Children's Food Trust began work as a non-departmental public body for the then Department of Education and Skills (replaced by the Department for Children, Schools and Families and subsequently by the current Department for Education (DfE). The Government announced new legal standards for school food in England in May 2006 and the Children's Food Trust was asked to lead their national implementation. The national standards now make sure that the average school lunch offers the right mix of energy and nutrients for growing children and limits their exposure to sugary, fatty, and salty foods. Since then, experts have advised Government at both national and local level on a wide range of other robust, but deliverable, ways of improving food in schools.

Care Quality Commission

The Care Quality Commission (CQC) checks all hospitals and care establishments in England to ensure they are meeting government standards and share the findings with the public via various reports.

Reader Reflections

Look at the eight tips on healthy eating. Do you achieve them all?

If you work in a care establishment, are they all achieved?

Have you seen information on nutrition and health from any of the organisations listed?

Sources of Nutrients

Fluid

Water makes up more than two thirds of human body weight and without water we would die in a few days. While it is not considered to be a nutrient, it is absolutely fundamental to life.

- The human brain is made up of 95% water
- Blood, which transports nutrients and other substances around the body, is 82% water
- Lungs are 90% water and have a moist membrane which helps to ward off infections
- Fluid is needed to keep the joints and muscles functioning
- Lack of fluid can also contribute to bowel problems such as constipation.

A mere 2% drop in our body's water supply can trigger signs of dehydration which include: fuzzy short-term memory, trouble with basic maths and difficulty focusing on smaller print, such as on a computer screen. Mild dehydration is also one of the most common causes of daytime fatigue. An estimated 75% of people have mild dehydration.

Fluid is lost from the body in the urine, exhaled air, faeces and perspiration. People working in hot environments and also those who are very active will require more.

Adults are advised to drink 1.5 - 2 litres (6-8 cups or glasses) per day. All fluids count especially water, juices, squashes, teas, coffees, milk and soft drinks. Alcohol and very strong caffeine drinks, for example an espresso, do not count as they act as diuretics stimulating the kidneys to pass more urine.

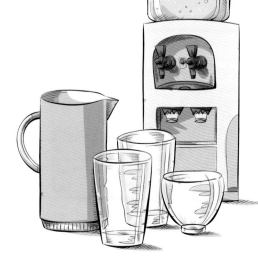

Alcohol

The majority of people in the UK drink alcohol at some time. It does not contribute to the fluid content of the diet.

Alcohol provides calories and can therefore contribute to obesity and also, in excess, to CHD (coronary heart disease)

A further concern about excessive alcohol consumption is that its contribution to liver disease, called cirrhosis, in which the liver first starts to develop fatty tissues and then ultimately scar tissue. This means the liver cannot undertake its normal functions.

The usual limits are regarded as women taking no more than 2-3 units per day and men 3-4 units per day. One alcohol unit is measured as 10ml or 8g of pure alcohol. This equals one 25ml single measure of whisky (ABV 40%), or a third of a pint of beer (ABV 5-6%) or half a standard (175ml) glass of red wine (ABV 12%).

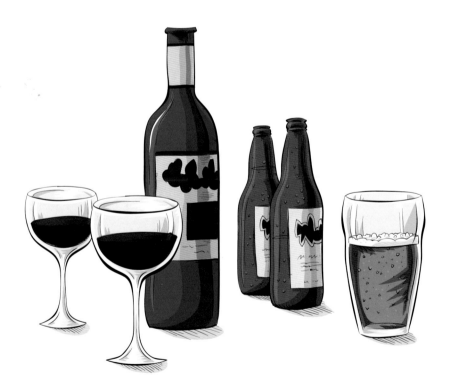

Energy

Energy is needed for the Basal Metabolic Rate (BMR) which is the rate the body uses energy for the functions that keep us alive such as keeping the heart beating, blood circulating and breathing. Activities also need energy and the more active a person is, the more energy they will need. Periods of growth during childhood and pregnancy require energy. Healing after wounds or illnesses also requires energy.

Energy is measured in kilocalories (kcal) often called calories and also kilojoules (kJ). Therefore food energy is also expressed in kilo calories (kcal) and kilojoules (kJ). Within the European Union, both the kilocalorie (kcal) and kilojoule (kJ) appear on food labels. In many countries, only one of the units is displayed.

Dietary Reference Values (DRVs)

In the UK, estimated requirements for various groups within the UK population were examined and published by the Committee on Medical Aspects of Food and Nutrition Policy (COMA) in the 1991 report 'Dietary Reference Values for Food Energy and Nutrients for the United Kingdom'. COMA has now been replaced by the Scientific Advisory Committee on Nutrition (SACN) who are likely to review the UK nutritional requirements in the near future. DRVs are a series of estimates of the amount of energy and nutrients needed by different groups of healthy people in the UK population; they are not recommendations or goals for individuals.

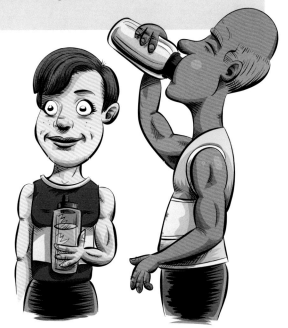

Estimated Average Requirements (EARs) are the figures used for energy and in the table below it can be seen that adults need more than children.

Guideline Daily Amounts (GDAs) are figures used for protein, vitamins and minerals.

Estimated Average Requirements (EARs) for Energy

Age		EARs MJ/day (kcal/day)			
		Males		Females	
0-3 months		2.28	545	2.16	(515)
4-6 month		2.89	690	2.69	(645)
7-9 months		3.44	825	3.20	(765)
10-12 months		3.85	920	3.61	(865)
1-3 years		5.15	1 230	4.86	(1 165)
4-6 years		7.16	1 715	6.46	(1 545)
7-10 years		8.24	1 970	7.28	(1 740)
11-14 years		9.27	2 220	7.72	(1 845)
15-18 years		11.51	2 755	8.83	(2 110)
19-50 years		10.60	2 550	8.10	(1 940)
51-59 years		10.60	2 550	8.00	(1 900)
60-64 years		9.93	2 380	7.99	(1 900)
65-74 years		9.71	2 330	7.96	(1 900)
75+		8.77	2 100	7.61	(1 810)
Pregnancy	(last 3 months only)			+0.8	(200)
Lactation	(0-1 months)			+1.9	(450)
	(1-2 month)			+2.2	(530)
	(2-3 months)			+2.4	(570)
Group 1*	(4-6 months)			+2.0	(480)
Group 2	(6+ months)			+1.0	(240)
Group 1*	(4-6 months)			+2.4	(570)
Group 2	(6+ months)			+2.3	(550)

* Women in group 1 progressively introduce weaning foods when the baby is 3-4 months. Women in Group 2 only introduce limited foods at this age and breast milk is still the main source of nourishment for the baby.

Men need more energy as they generally have a larger body size, more muscle and are more active.

	Calories
Women	2000
Men	2500
Children 5–10	1800

Excess energy intake leads to excess energy from food being converted to fat and deposited in the body, leading to weight increase and obesity. And if someone takes in inadequate energy they lose weight as they burn up the body's deposits of fat. This can result in malnourishment.

Food Labels and Nutrients
Some food labels use a traffic light colour coding system. This indicates whether the food has high(red), medium(amber) or low(groon) amounts of fat, saturated fat, sugars and salt.

- A high amount of sugar is more than 15g per 100g and
- A low amount of sugar is 5g per 100g
- A high amount of fat is more than 20g per 100g and
- A low amount of fat is 3g per 100g
- A high amount of saturated fat is is more than 5g per 100g and
- A low amount of saturated fat is 1.5g per 100g
- A high amount of salt is more than 1.5g per 100g (0.6g sodium) and
- A low amount of salt is 0.3g per 100g (0.1g sodium).

Different nutrients provide different amounts of energy, with fat providing the most energy. Energy from nutrients (kcal/calories per gram):

- Carbohydrate 3.75
- Protein 4
- Fat 9
- Alcohol 7

Looking at the total diet and energy requirements, it is considered that carbohydrate is the preferred source for energy and the following percentages of the total dietary energy should be used.

- 50% energy from carbohydrate
  (10% from sugars)
- 30-35% from fats

Carbohydrates
As already seen, carbohydrate is the major source of energy. There are three major groups of carbohydrates:

- Sugars
- Starches
- Fibre or non-starch polysaccharide (NSP).

Both sugars and starches provide 3.75 kcal per gram, but fibre cannot be used for energy to any significant extent.

Sugars

All sugars can cause tooth decay. Many processed foods contain sugar and the higher it appears in the list of ingredients, the more sugar there is in the product. When reading the labels remember that 'no added sugar' does not necessarily mean that the product is sugar free. It simply means that no extra sugar has been added.

Tooth decay or dental caries is one of the most common of all disorders. It usually occurs in children and young adults but can affect any person. It is a common cause of tooth loss in younger people. Bacteria are normally present in the mouth and convert all foods, especially sugar, into acids. Bacteria, acid, food debris and saliva combine in the mouth to form a sticky substance called plaque that adheres to the teeth. It is most prominent on the back molars, just above the gum line on all teeth, and at the edges of fillings. Plaque that is not removed from the teeth mineralises into tartar. Plaque and tartar irritate the gums. Plaque begins to build up on teeth within 20 minutes after eating (the time when most bacterial activity occurs). If this plaque is not removed thoroughly and routinely, tooth decay will not only begin, but flourish. The acids in plaque dissolve the enamel surface of the tooth and create holes in the tooth called cavities. Cavities are usually painless until they grow very large and affect nerves or cause a tooth fracture.

Sugars increase the risk of tooth decay. Sticky foods are more harmful than nonsticky foods because they remain on the surface of the teeth. Frequent snacking increases the time that acids are in contact with the surface of the tooth.

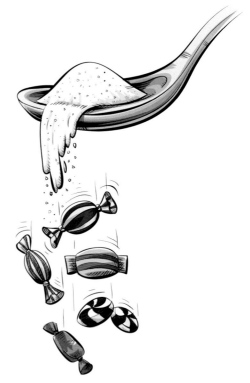

Added sugars are called extrinsic sugars and are the type most likely to cause dental problems. This sugar is usually table sugar, which is called sucrose and is found in sweets and soft drinks as well as cakes and pastries. Pure sugar has no other nutrients in it.

The Children's Food Trust has standards for the maximum amount of extrinsic sugar in school lunches.

Intrinsic sugar is natural sugar and is found inside fruit (e.g. apples, oranges, peaches) and vegetables (e.g. carrots, parsnips, tomatoes).

Monosaccharides and Disaccharides

Glucose, galactose, and fructose are 'single' sugars or monosaccharides. Two monosaccharides can be linked together to form a 'double' sugar or disaccharide. When carbohydrates are eaten they are broken down in the process of digestion into monosacchrides, which can then be absorbed into the bloodstream and used for energy.

- **Glucose**, 'blood sugar', the immediate source of energy cells
- **Galactose**, a sugar in milk and yoghurt
- **Fructose**, a sugar found in fruit and honey

Three common disaccharides:

- **Sucrose**, common table sugar – glucose + fructose
- **Lactose**, major sugar in milk = glucose + galactose
- **Maltose**, product of starch digestion = glucose + glucose

Some people cannot break down the disaccharide lactose during the process of digestion and are said to be intolerant of it.

Starchy Foods

These foods contain starches also known as polysaccharides. Usually they are also associated with other nutrients like B vitamins, iron and protein. Unrefined starchy foods also contain fibre.

Starchy foods such as potatoes, bread, cereals, rice and pasta should make up about a third of the food you eat. Where you can, choose wholegrain varieties which also contain fibre. Starch is the most common form of carbohydrate in our diet and some starchy foods should be eaten every day as part of a healthy balanced diet. Data published by the National Diet and Nutrition Survey, which looks at food consumption in the UK, shows that most of us should be eating more starchy foods.

Starchy foods are a good source of energy and the main source of a range of nutrients in our diet.

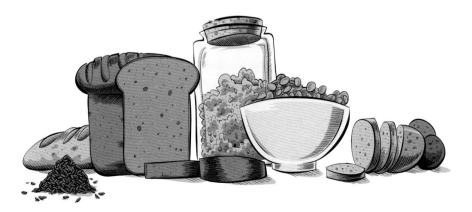

Fibre

Fibre (which used to be called roughage) or non-starch polysaccharide (NSP) helps to keep the bowel regular as well as to prevent bowel cancer. Foods containing lots of fibre fill us up for longer, so we're much less likely to overeat.

People should eat 18-24g of fibre per day but most people only eat about 12g per day, which can contribute to bowel problems like constipation, bowel cancer and haemorrhoids (piles). For this reason people are encouraged to eat more fibre.

Sources of fibre include wholegrain breakfast cereals (Weetabix, branflakes, unsweetened muesli, Shreddies and porridge oats), wholemeal pasta, brown rice, pulses, nuts and seeds. Vegetables and fruit are also a source of fibre, especially when the skins are eaten.

Fibre has many uses in the body, as well as providing 'roughage' to prevent constipation. Lack of fibre is thought to be connected with various disorders of the bowel, including a serious inflammation called diverticulitis. Fibre also slows down digestion. Soluble fibre, such as that in beans and lentils controls blood sugar more effectively than insoluble fibre and may also lower blood cholesterol, if high. Insoluble fibre such as wheat bran soaks up water thus providing bulk, which causes waste to be passed more quickly through the gut and also gives the feeling of being full. Eating more fibre may actually help people to stay slim. Food with plenty of fibre such as potatoes and bread can be satisfying without providing too many calories.

Fats

Fats provide the highest source of calories for energy (9kcal/g). Some fat is needed in the body for insulation under the skin and as protection around the vital organs. It is found in part of the nervous tissue and brain and also acts as an energy store in the body.

Obesity

This is due to an excess store of fat which can be particularly harmful if deposited around the middle area of the body. Deposits of fat around the waist and stomach, the so called 'apple shape', are linked with CHD, Type 2 diabetes and high blood pressure.

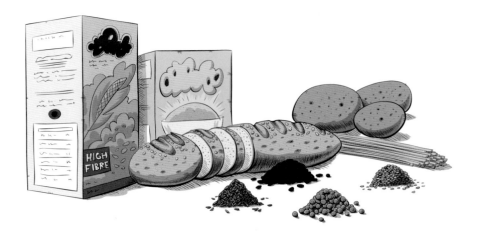

Saturated Fat

Eating a diet that is high in saturated fat can raise the level of bad cholesterol in the blood. High cholesterol increases the risk of heart disease. Most people eat too much saturated fat; about 20% more than the recommended maximum amount.

- The average man should eat no more than 30g of saturated fat a day.
- The average woman should eat no more than 20g of saturated fat a day.

Foods containing saturated fat are:

- Butter and hard margarine as well as items containing them such as cakes and biscuits
- Lard and items like pastries and pies
- Hard cheese such as Cheddar or Red Leicester
- Coconut oil and cream such as in korma dishes
- Palm oil and dishes and products with it in.

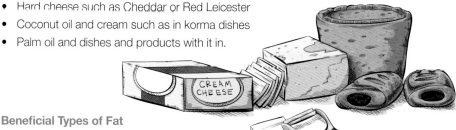

Beneficial Types of Fat

Unsaturated fats are the beneficial ones as they help to prevent CHD. They include monounsaturated fat and polyunsaturated fat.

Monounsaturated fats are found in rapeseed oil, olive oil, avocado oil and groundnut oil as well as spreads made from them. Polyunsaturated fats are found in soya oil, corn oil and sunflower oils, as well as in spreads made from them.

Omega 3 Fats

These are unsaturated fats which are needed for healthy brain function and also help to prevent CHD.

Sources of omega 3 fatty acids are oily fish, which are:

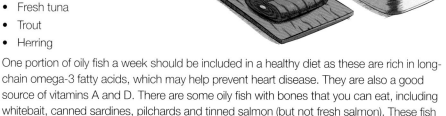

- Mackerel
- Salmon
- Sardines
- Pilchards
- Fresh tuna
- Trout
- Herring

One portion of oily fish a week should be included in a healthy diet as these are rich in long-chain omega-3 fatty acids, which may help prevent heart disease. They are also a good source of vitamins A and D. There are some oily fish with bones that you can eat, including whitebait, canned sardines, pilchards and tinned salmon (but not fresh salmon). These fish can help strengthen bones because they are good sources of calcium and phosphorus.

Proteins

Proteins are the major functional and structural components of all the cells of the body and they are essential for their growth and repair. All enzymes, blood transport molecules, antibodies, hair, fingernails and many hormones are proteins. Proteins are made of sequences of amino acids linked together.

Each gram of protein provides 4 calories and can therefore be used as a source of energy. However, the body prefers using carbohydrates and fats as its first source of energy. Proteins are found in different foods. Some animal sources of proteins are meat, poultry, fish, eggs, milk, cheese and yogurt. Plant sources of proteins include legumes (or pulses such as beans and lentils), grains, nuts, seeds and cereals. Proteins should contribute 10-15% of our total energy (calorie) intake. This amount is essential to maintain the required protein turnover necessary for the normal growth and repair of body tissues. It is also important to introduce proteins into our diet because we cannot produce all the amino acids we need. Therefore we must get 'essential amino-acids' from food.

The Guideline Daily Amount (GDA) for proteins is 45g for women and 55g for men.

Amino Acids

These are the building blocks of protein; some amino acids are called essential or indispensable which means they cannot be made by the body. There are also non-essential (dispensable) amino acids which can be made by the body from other amino acids. Eggs, meat and fish are good sources of all the essential (indispensable) amino acids.

Vitamins and Minerals

These are vital for body functions and are called micronutrients as they are needed in tiny amounts. Most people should be able to get all the nutrients they need by eating a balanced diet There are two types of vitamins: fat-soluble and water-soluble.

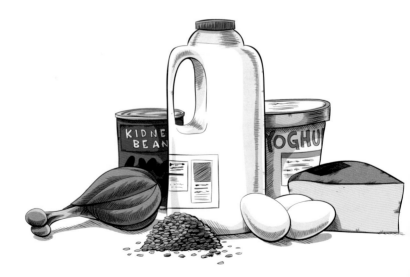

Fat-Soluble Vitamins

Fat-soluble vitamins are found mainly in fatty foods such as animal fats including butter and lard, vegetable oils, dairy foods, liver and oily fish. While the body needs these vitamins every day to work properly, you do not need to eat foods containing them every day. If the body does not need these vitamins immediately, it stores them in your liver and fatty tissues for future use. These stores can build up so they are there when needed. However, large amounts of fat-soluble vitamins can be harmful.

Fat-soluble vitamins are:

- Vitamin A
- Vitamin D
- Vitamin E
- Vitamin K

Water-Soluble Vitamins

Water-soluble vitamins are not stored in the body, therefore you need to eat foods containing these vitamins more frequently. If excess is taken, the body gets rid of the extra vitamins in the urine. Because the body does not store water-soluble vitamins, these vitamins are generally not harmful. Water-soluble vitamins are found in fruit, vegetables and grains. Unlike fat-soluble vitamins, they can be destroyed by heat or by being exposed to air.

They can also be lost in water used for cooking. This means that by cooking foods, especially boiling them, we lose many of these vitamins. The best way to keep as much of the water-soluble vitamins as possible is to steam or grill these foods, rather than boil them.

Water-soluble vitamins:

- Vitamin C
- B vitamin group, folic acid and also vitamin B12

Vitamin A

This is required for eyesight and the immune function. It is found in fatty foods such as:

- Oily fish
- Butter, margarine
- Egg yolk
- Full fat milk
- Liver

Excess vitamin A should not be taken in pregnancy as it is harmful. Liver is not recommended as fat-soluble vitamins are stored in the liver.

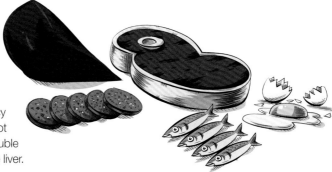

Vitamin A can be made in the body from the precursor called Beta Carotene (which acts as a protective antioxidant itself). Beta Carotene is found in orange-red coloured foods such as carrots, apricots, mangoes and also green vegetables.

Vitamin D

This vitamin aids calcium absorption and thus helps with the development of the skeleton. A lack causes rickets in children or osteomalacia in adults, although rickets occurs rarely now. We can make vitamin D by the action of sunlight on the skin.

Food sources of vitamin D include:

- Oily fish
- Butter, margarine
- Egg yolk
- Full fat milk
- Liver

People who are at risk of a deficiency are those who cover themselves from the sunlight and those who do not go outside very much.

It is recommended that people over 65 years who do not eat foods containing vitamin D should take a supplement. This helps to keep bones strong thus reducing the frequency of falls.

Vitamin E

This is an antioxidant, which is important to heart health.

Sources of vitamin E are:

- Nuts
- Seeds
- Wholegrains

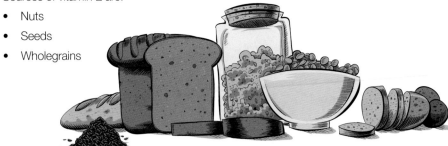

Vitamin K

This vitamin is particularly important in helping blood to clot. It also has a role in the skeleton. Green vegetables like cabbage, sprouts and beans are good sources. Vitamin K is made by bacteria in the bowel. Newborn babies have a sterile gut so they have no bacteria to make vitamin K and thus need a supplement.

B Vitamin Group

The B vitamins are all water soluble and are generally used for energy release from foods in cells. Vitamin B12 is needed for blood cell formation and Folate (which is the natural form of the vitamin) for the nervous system.

Sources of most B vitamins are:

- Wholegrains
- Meat
- Dairy products
- Fortified breakfast cereals
- Yeast extracts

Vitamin B12 is found mainly in foods of animal origin so those who do not eat animal products, such as vegans, can develop a type of anaemia from a deficiency. It is important that they ensure they have a source from a supplement or from items like soya milk with added vitamin B12.

Sources of vitamin B12 are:

- Meat and fish
- Dairy products
- Fortified breakfast cereals
- Yeast extracts

Folate is needed for the nervous tissue and blood cells. Folate is the natural source found in foods and folic acid is the supplement. During the first 12 weeks of pregnancy a supplement of folic acid is advised. This helps to prevent neural tube defects like spina bifida. A supplement of folic acid is also recommended for any woman who wishes to become pregnant.

Folate sources are:

- Fortified breakfast cereals
- Wholegrains
- Beans of all types
- Green vegetables
- Yeast extracts

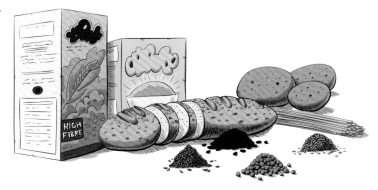

Vitamin C

Vitamin C helps to keep skin and tissues, as well as blood vessel walls, healthy and also aids iron absorption. Vitamin C is an antioxidant and is therefore protective for the immune system. Severe deficiency can lead to scurvy. Vitamin C is easily destroyed in cooking. To avoid some of the vitamin loss in cooking do not peel or chop fruit and vegetables finely. Do not overcook them or keep them warm for long periods after cooking and cook in a minimum amount of water. Freezing locks in the vitamins, so frozen vegetables are a good source of vitamin C.

Vitamin C sources are:

- Citrus fruit
- Potatoes
- Green vegetables
- Berries
- Salads

Minerals

Minerals are necessary for three main reasons:

- Building strong bones and teeth
- Controlling body fluids inside and outside cells
- Ensuring the formation of haemoglobin in blood

Minerals are found in varying amounts in foods such as meat, cereals (including cereal products such as bread) fish, milk and dairy foods, vegetables, fruit (especially dried fruit) and nuts.

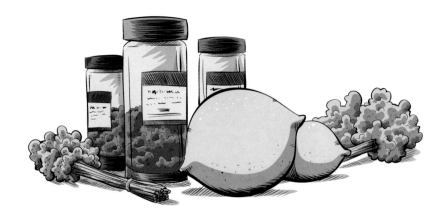

Calcium

Calcium has several important functions including helping to build strong bones and teeth, regulating muscle contractions such as the heartbeat and ensuring blood clots normally.

It is thought that calcium may help lower high blood pressure. A lack of calcium can lead to a condition called rickets in children and osteomalacia in adults. Adequate calcium and good skeletal development assists in preventing osteoporosis in later life. Vitamin D is needed for calcium absorption. Teenagers, pregnant women and breastfeeding women have a greater requirement for calcium.

Good sources of calcium include:

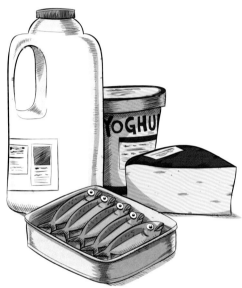

- Milk, cheese and other dairy foods such as yoghurt

- Green leafy vegetables such as broccoli, cabbage and okra, but not spinach

- Soya beans

- Tofu and soya drinks with added calcium

- Nuts

- Bread and foods made with fortified flour

- Fish with edible bones, such as sardines and pilchards

Iron

Iron is an essential mineral that has several important roles in the body. It helps make red blood cells which carry oxygen around the body. A lack of iron can lead to iron deficiency anaemia; symptoms of this include tiredness, paleness, breathlessness and poor wound healing. Women of childbearing age need more iron due to the monthly blood loss. Older people can lack iron, as they may not eat foods containing iron if they have dental problems. They may also be on medication that interferes with the absorption of iron. As they do not eat meat, which provides an easily absorbed source of iron, vegetarians and vegans can lack iron if their diet is not carefully balanced.

Many people think that spinach is a good source of iron, however, spinach also contains a substance that makes it harder for the body to absorb the iron from it. Similarly, tea and coffee contain a substance that can make it harder for the body to absorb iron which is why cutting down on tea and coffee could help improve your iron levels. Vitamin C also aids the absorption of iron.

Good sources of iron include:

- Liver
- Meat
- Beans
- Nuts
- Dried fruit, such as dried apricots
- Wholegrains, such as brown rice
- Fortified breakfast cereals
- Soybean flour
- Most dark-green leafy vegetables, such as watercress and curly kale

The iron in meat and offal, dark fish and poultry is called haem iron and is easily absorbed while that in vegetables, fruit and cereals is in the non-haem form which is poorly absorbed.

Sodium and Potassium

These two minerals are called electrolytes, as they are responsible for the fluid balance of the body and nervous and muscle impulses.

A diet that is high in salt (which contains sodium and is also called sodium chloride) can cause raised blood pressure, which around one third of adults in the UK already have. High blood pressure often has no symptoms. Those who have high blood pressure (hypertension) are more likely to develop heart disease or have a stroke. Cutting down on salt reduces blood pressure, which means that the risk of developing stroke or heart disease is reduced. We are advised not to have more than 6g of salt per day. On food labels salt is often named as sodium. To find out the amount of salt, multiply the amount of sodium by 2.5.

Sodium sources include:

- Processed foods
- Soups
- Ready meals
- Convenience foods
- Savoury snacks
- Bacon and ham
- Cheese
- Table salt

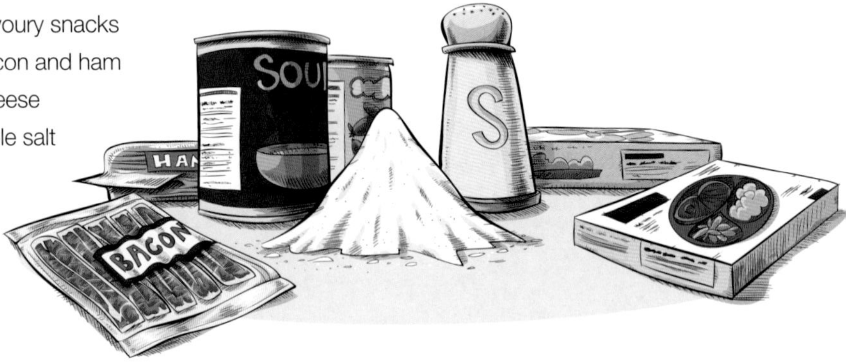

Most sodium is derived from processed foods. On food labels a high amount of salt is more than 1.5g per 100g (0.6g sodium), and a low amount of salt is 0.3g per 100g (0.1g sodium)

Potassium is also an electrolyte and works in balance with sodium. Potassium is involved in the energy release system, which occurs in every cell of the body.

Potassium sources are:

- Fruit, especially bananas which are the richest source of potassium
- Vegetables

Reader Reflections

Consider the amount of carbohydrate that you eat. Could you choose more high fibre sources?

List the food sources of vitamin D and discuss who may lack this vitamin.

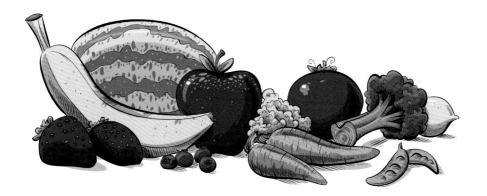

The eatwell plate

Use the eatwell plate to help you get the balance right. It shows how
much of what you eat should come from each food group.

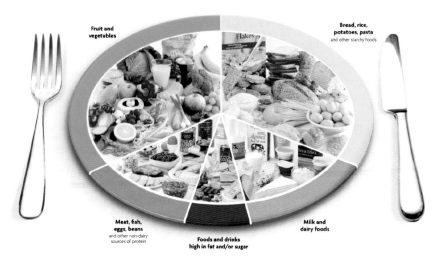

Fruit and
vegetables

Bread, rice,
potatoes, pasta
and other starchy foods

Meat, fish,
eggs, beans
and other non-dairy
sources of protein

Foods and drinks
high in fat and/or sugar

Milk and
dairy foods

Department of Health in association with the Welsh Assembly Government, the Scottish Government and the Food Standards Agency in Northern Ireland

Diet and Health

Eatwell Plate

The eatwell plate shows government guidelines for the different types of food we need to
eat, and in what proportions, to have a well balanced and healthy diet. The eatwell plate
applies to most people, whether they are a healthy weight or overweight, on a low fat diet,
have diabetes, whether they eat meat or are vegetarian, and no matter what their ethnic
origin. There is great emphasis on variety to ensure we get a full range of nutrients.

However the eatwell plate does not apply to children under the age of two because
they have different nutritional needs. Between the ages of two and five, children should
gradually move to eating the same foods as the rest of the family, in the proportions shown
on the eatwell plate. Anyone with special dietary requirements or medical needs might
want to check with a registered dietitian or registered nutritionist whether the eatwell plate
applies to them.

There are five segments in the eatwell plate and the two largest segments are fruit
and vegetables and bread, rice, potatoes, pasta, breakfast cereals and other starchy
carbohydrates. The smallest is foods and drinks high in fats and/or sugars, which are the
least healthy group.

It should be remembered that there are no bad foods, only bad diets with excessive
amounts of foods and drinks high in fats and/or sugars and too little fruit and vegetables.

The segments in the eatwell plate are as follows:

Bread, Rice, Potatoes, Pasta and Other Starchy Foods

We should eat plenty of potatoes, bread, rice, pasta and other starchy foods and ideally wholegrain varieties should be eaten as they have more fibre. This group is the main source of starchy carbohydrates which is needed for energy plus B vitamins, some iron and calcium.

Fruit and Vegetables

We should also eat plenty of fruit and vegetables. The 5 A DAY programme highlights the health benefits of getting five 80g portions of fruit and vegetables every day. This means five portions of fruit and vegetables altogether, not five portions of each.

- There are many types of fruit and vegetables to choose from, which makes it easy to eat a variety.
- They are a good source of vitamins and minerals, including folate, vitamin C and potassium
- They are an excellent source of dietary fibre, which helps maintain a healthy gut and prevent constipation and other digestion problems. A diet high in fibre can also reduce the risk of bowel cancer
- They contain antioxidants which can help reduce the risk of heart disease, stroke and some cancers
- Fruit and vegetables contribute to a healthy and balanced diet.

Fruit and vegetables are also usually low in fat and calories (provided you don't fry or roast them in lots of oil) That's why eating them can help maintain a healthy weight and keep the heart healthy.

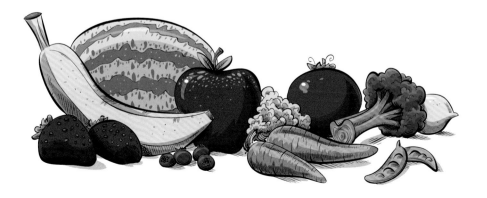

Milk and Dairy Foods

Milk and dairy products such as cheese and yoghurt are good sources of protein and calcium. Our bodies need protein to work properly and to grow or repair themselves. Calcium helps to keep our bones strong. The calcium in dairy foods is particularly good because the body absorbs it easily. Choose lower-fat dairy foods where possible, because these are healthier choices. The total fat content of dairy products can vary a lot. Fat in milk provides calories for young children and also contains essential vitamins such as vitamins A and D. Soya milk is also included in this group and is useful for those who cannot tolerate cow's milk.

- Full cream (whole milk) contains fat and vitamins A and D
- Semi-skimmed milk has half of the fat remaining and most of the vitamins A and D removed
- Fully skimmed milk has fat and vitamins A and D removed.

Meat, Fish, Eggs, Beans and Other Non-Dairy Sources of Protein

This group provides protein, B vitamins, iron and minerals. A balanced diet can include protein from meat, as well as from non-animal sources such as beans and pulses.

Meat is a good source of protein in the diet, as well as vitamins and minerals. Some meats are high in saturated fat, which can raise blood cholesterol levels. It is recommended that you only eat a small amount of red and processed meat due to the fat and salt these contain. Meats such as chicken, pork, lamb and beef are all rich in protein. Red meat is a good source of iron, and meat is also one of the main sources of vitamin B12.

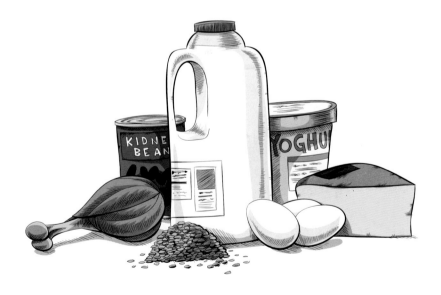

Fish is a source of protein, iron and B vitamins. White fish such as cod or plaice is low in fat. Oily fish provides Omega 3 fatty acids plus vitamins A and D. If the bones are eaten, calcium is also provided.

Poultry such as chicken and turkey is a source of protein, iron and B vitamins. It is also low in fat as long as the skin is not eaten.

Eggs are a good choice as part of a healthy, balanced diet. As well as being a source of protein, they also contain vitamins and minerals including vitamin D, vitamin A and iron. They can be part of a healthy meal that's quick and easy to make.

There is no recommended limit on how many eggs people should eat. However, to get the nutrients you need, make sure you eat as varied a diet as possible. Eggs contain cholesterol and high cholesterol levels in our blood increase our risk of heart disease. However, the cholesterol we get from food, including eggs, has less effect on the amount of cholesterol in our blood than the amount of saturated fat we eat.

Pulses are a cheap, low-fat source of protein, fibre, vitamins and minerals, and they count towards your recommended five daily portions of fruit and vegetables. A pulse is an edible seed that grows in a pod.

Pulses include all beans, peas and lentils, such as:

- Baked beans
- Red, green, yellow and brown lentils
- Black-eyed peas
- Garden peas
- Chickpeas
- Broad beans
- Kidney beans
- Butter beans

Pulses are a source of protein. This means they can be particularly important for people who do not get protein by eating meat, fish or dairy products. Pulses can also be a healthy, low fat choice for meat eaters. You can add pulses to soups, casseroles and meat sauces to add extra texture and flavour. Pulses are a good source of iron, they are also a starchy food and add fibre to your meal. The fibre found in pulses may help lower blood cholesterol, so they are good for your heart. Pulses count as one of the five recommended daily portions of fruit and vegetables. One portion is three heaped tablespoons of cooked pulses.

Foods and Drinks High in Fat and/or Sugar

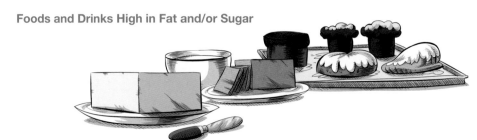

Eating too much fat can cause weight gain because foods that are high in fat are also high in energy (calories). Being overweight raises our risk of serious health problems, such as heart disease, Type 2 diabetes and high blood pressure.
But this doesn't mean that all fat is bad. We need some fat in our diet because it helps the body absorb certain nutrients such as fat soluble vitamins. Fat is a source of energy, and provides essential fatty acids that the body can't make itself. Unsaturated fats are better for our health.

Most adults and children in the UK eat too much sugar. Sugars occur naturally in foods such as fruit and milk, but we do not need to cut down on these types of sugars. The sugar we should cut down on is the type added to a wide range of foods, such as sweets, cakes, biscuits, chocolate, and some fizzy drinks and juice drinks.

Fast Foods and Convenience Foods

These foods are quick and easy to purchase and tend to be a uniform cost and recipe wherever they are bought. They may be useful at times when people are travelling or in a rush. However they are often:

- High in fat
- High in saturated fat
- High in salt
- Low in fibre
- Low in fruit and vegetables

They also contain additives.

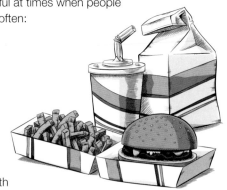

Reader Reflections

Consider the food you eat or serve in line with those in the eatwell plate.

Do you eat or serve five portions of fruit and vegetables per day? If not, how can this be increased?

Special Diets

Benefits of a Healthy Diet and Effects of an Unhealthy Diet

Eating a well balanced diet can help people not only to feel well and look better, but to assist in preventing various health problems. For children a healthy diet assists with correct growth. For those who develop health problems like obesity, adherence to an appropriate diet can help to manage the problem.

Problems associated with an unhealthy diet include:

- Obesity
- Dental decay (caries)
- High blood pressure, strokes
- Type 2 diabetes
- Constipation
- Cancer
- Coronary Heart disease (CHD)

Obesity occurs when a person is carrying too much body fat for their height and sex. A person is considered obese if they have a body mass index (BMI) of 30 or greater. Today's way of life is less physically active than it used to be. People travel on buses and

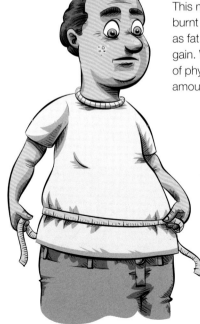

in cars, rather than walking, and many people work in offices, where they are sitting still for most of the day. This means that the calories they eat are not getting burnt off as energy. Instead, the extra calories are stored as fat. Over time, eating excess calories leads to weight gain. Without lifestyle changes to increase the amount of physical activity done on a daily basis, or reduce the amount of calories consumed, people can become obese.

In 2008, nearly a quarter of adults (those over 16 years of age) in England were obese (had a BMI over 30). Just under a third of women, 32%, and 42% of men were overweight (a BMI of 25-30). Amongst children (2 –15 years of age), one in six boys and one in seven girls in England were obese in 2008. The number of overweight and obese people is likely to increase.

The Foresight report, a scientific report used to guide government policy, has predicted that by 2025 nearly half of men and over a third of women will be obese.

High blood pressure is known as the 'silent killer' and rarely has obvious symptoms. Around 30% of people in England have high blood pressure but many do not know it. If left untreated, high blood pressure increases your risk of a heart attack or stroke.

Diabetes develops when the body does not produce enough insulin to maintain a normal blood glucose level, or when the body is unable to effectively use the insulin that is being produced. Type 2 diabetes is the most common form of diabetes and usually occurs in older and often overweight individuals.

Constipation is a very common condition that affects people of all ages. It can mean stools (faeces) are not passed as often as normal.

Cancers come in many different types and are a group of conditions in which the body's cells begin to grow and reproduce in an uncontrollable way. These cells can then invade and destroy healthy tissue, including organs. Cancer sometimes begins in one part of the body before spreading to other parts. This process is known as metastasis. Changes to lifestyle can significantly reduce the risk of developing cancer, for example, eating a healthy diet, taking regular exercise and avoiding smoking.

Coronary heart disease (CHD) is the UK's biggest killer. Around one in five men and one in seven women die from the disease. CHD causes around 94,000 deaths in the UK each year. CHD affects more men than women, and the chance of getting it increases with age. The heart is a muscle that is about the size of a fist. It pumps blood around your body and beats approximately 70 times a minute. After the blood leaves the right side of the heart, it goes to your lungs where it picks up oxygen. The oxygen-rich blood returns to your heart and is then pumped to the organs of your body through a network of arteries. The blood returns to your heart through veins before being pumped back to your lungs again. This process is called circulation. The heart gets its own supply of blood from a network of blood vessels on the surface of your heart, called coronary arteries. Coronary heart disease is the term that describes what happens when your heart's blood supply is blocked or interrupted by a build-up of fatty substances in the coronary arteries.

Special Diets

There are a number of conditions that are assisted by special or therapeutic diets and Registered Dietitians are able to assist with advising on a correct diet. The following diets are commonly used to assist people:

- Low calorie/slimming diets for those who are overweight or obese
- Diets for those who are diabetic
- Diets for people with allergies and intolerances of various types
- Diets for those who are malnourished or who are underweight and have deficiencies
- Vegetarian and vegan diets
- Religious diets

Overweight and Obesity

This is a major problem. According to the Foresight report, about 50% of the adult population and 20% of children are overweight or obese. It is a complex disorder due to too many calories (energy) being eaten in excess of needs for the BMR (Basal Metabolic Rate) and level of activity. Often an excess of fatty and sugary foods as well as alcohol may have been consumed. Also, a lack of exercise contributes to the development of obesity. Obesity contributes to the development of:

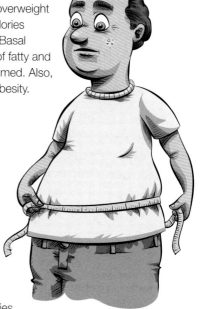

- Type 2 diabetes
- CHD
- Cancer
- High blood pressure

Diets for anyone who is overweight or obese should ideally be based on the eatwell plate with calorie intake reduced by about 500 per day to ensure a slow steady weight loss of about half a kilo per week. Snacks should be swapped for something healthier and include more fruit and vegeatables. Many common snacks, such as sweets, chocolate, biscuits and crisps, are high in fat and sugar and calories that we do not need. Elevenses or typical mid-afternoon snacks can be swapped for a piece of fruit, a fruit bun or a slice of malt loaf with a low-fat spread. Meals should be based on starchy carbohydrates but not on types that are prepared with fats, such as chips.

Drinks that are high in calories should be swapped for drinks that are lower in fat and sugars. Swap a sugary, fizzy drink for a sparkling water or low calorie drink with a slice of lemon. Alcohol is also high in calories, so cutting down could help control weight.

Obesity is often measured by the BMI (Body Mass Index) which is a measure of weight in relation to height and the various figures give an indication of a healthy weight.

Diabetes

Diabetes affects over two million people in the UK. There are two types of diabetes Type1 diabetes affects younger people and requires insulin for its management and Type 2 diabetes affects older people and is often linked with being overweight. It may be managed by diet or diet plus tablets and occasionally by insulin. Type 2 diabetes is the more common type and affects 85% of those with diabetes.

Diabetes occurs when the glucose produced by eating carbohydrates cannot be used by the body for energy purposes due to a lack of the hormone insulin. This hormone is produced by the pancreas and allows cells to take up glucose. In Type I diabetes the insulin secretion stops entirely but in Type 2 diabetes the insulin is not adequate or effective.

Symptoms include thirst, tiredness, passing extra urine and raised blood glucose (sugar) levels.

People with diabetes should aim for normal blood glucose (sugar) levels, a normal weight and the avoidance of complications by having regular checks.

A healthy diet aims to ensure that people:

- Eat regular meals including breakfast
- Eat a balanced diet by following the eatwell plate
- Ensure that some starchy carbohydrate is eaten at each meal. Choose wholemeal, wholegrain, brown or granary products and foods with a lower glycaemic index such as pulses and oats
- Avoid excess added sugar by not adding extra sugar to cereals and drinks
- Avoid saturated fat and extra salt
- Aim for a normal weight.

The eatwell plate

Use the eatwell plate to help you get the balance right. It shows how much of what you eat should come from each food group.

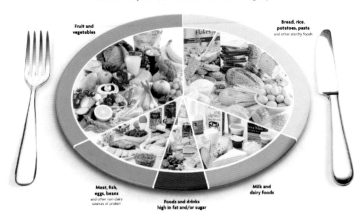

Department of Health in association with the Welsh Assembly Government, the Scottish Government and the Food Standards Agency in Northern Ireland

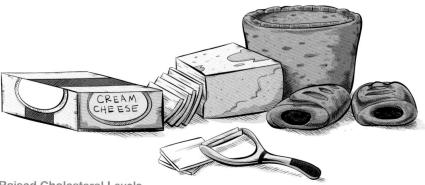

Raised Cholesterol Levels

Too much cholesterol can block the arteries in the heart causing a heart attack and CHD. A healthy diet should be balanced with regular meals and follow the eatwell plate. Avoid saturated fats and use monounsaturated fat instead for cooking and in spreads. Hard cheeses like cheddar cheese should only be used in small amounts with edam or cottage cheese being selected in preference. Choosing wholemeal, wholegrain, brown or granary products and oat based cereals assists in reducing cholesterol levels. Eat at least five portions of fruit and vegetables a day and include oily fish as this helps to prevent CHD.

Raised Blood Pressure

This is also called hypertension and can be alleviated by reducing weight, if overweight, to a normal level. Avoid added salt and salty foods like crisps, salted nuts, bacon and ham and aim for no more than 6g of salt per day. Add flavour to cooking by using herbs and spices instead of salt. Check food labels for low levels of salt ie. 0.3g salt (0.1g sodium) per 100g.

Allergies and Intolerances

These can be extremely serious as people can suffer from anaphylactic shock in response to a food they are allergic to. Nut allergies are particularly likely to cause such symptoms. If someone suffers from an allergy or intolerance, careful checking of ingredients in dishes and food products is vital.

The following allergens are seen on food labels:

- Peanuts/groundnuts
- Crustaceans such as crabs
- Eggs
- Gluten
- Citrus
- Sunflower
- Soya beans (in milks, breads, tofu and TVP)
- Lupins (a source of protein)
- Sulphites over 10ppm
- Tree nuts such as hazelnuts
- Molluscs such as welks
- Milk and lactose
- Wheat
- Sesame
- Poppy seeds
- Celery and celeriac
- Mustard (seeds and oils)

Coeliac Disease

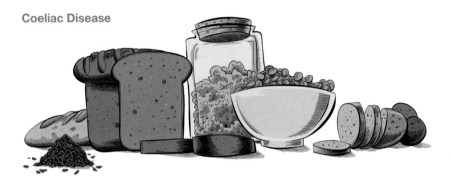

Coeliac disease is not an allergy or simple food intolerance. It is relatively common in the UK and is an autoimmune disease, where the body's immune system attacks its own tissues. In people with coeliac disease this immune reaction is triggered by gluten, a name for a type of protein found in the cereals wheat, rye and barley. A few people are also sensitive to oats.

People with undiagnosed coeliac disease suffer from various digestive problems including malabsorption, pain and discomfort. Those who have coeliac disease can have special gluten free products prescribed by their doctor and gluten free products are widely available.

Malnourishment

Older people and those who are sick or have had an operation or accident may become malnourished and loose significant amounts of weight. They require a high calorie high protein diet. Screening for malnutrition in all hospitals and care settings is recommended. One of the tools used for such screening is the MUST tool (Malnutrition Universal Screening Tool).

Vegetarians

The correct name for vegetarians is lacto–ovo vegetarians and this means that they:

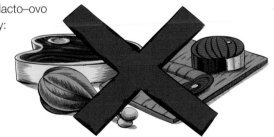

- Do not eat meat or poultry or products made from them
- Do not eat fish
- Do eat and drink milk and milk products
- Do eat eggs

Some people are lacto-vegetarian, which means as well as excluding meat, poultry and fish they also do not eat eggs. Some people are ovo-vegetarian, which means as well as excluding meat, poultry and fish they also do not eat or drink milk but do eat eggs. Omnivores are people who eat a diet including meat, fish and dairy products.

Vegans

Vegans exclude meat, poultry and fish as well as products derived from living creatures such as milk, eggs and honey. The restrictions mean that they can lack calcium, iron, protein and vitamin B12. To balance the diet vegans should include:

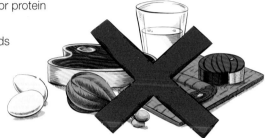

- Pulses and cereals for protein and iron
- Nuts, pulses, cereals and seeds for protein and iron
- Fruit and vegetables (vitamin C aids iron absorption)
- Fortified cereals or yeast extract for vitamin B12
- Soya milk with added calcium.

Religious Diets

Muslims

Muslims follow the Koran and do not eat pork or products derived from it. All meat and poultry must be Halal, which means it is killed in accordance with Islamic religious laws. They do not eat shellfish or drink alcohol.

Hindus

Hindus are often vegetarian and do not eat beef or products made from it such as burgers, as cattle are believed to be sacred. They do not usually drink alcohol.

Jewish Faith

Jewish people do not eat pork or pork products and they also do not have meat and milk at the same meal. Fish without fins and scales are not eaten.

Fasting

Some religions have periods of fasting. Muslims fast during the month of Ramadan. Hindus fast at various times and Christians observe Lent by giving up certain foods.

Reader Reflection

What would you have to consider when preparing food for someone with an intolerance to gluten and what would you check for on food labels?

Nutrition and Life Stages

Babies, Children and Teenagers

Babies

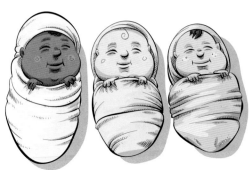

Breast milk (Colostrum) is perfectly and uniquely made for babies growing needs and giving them breastmilk can contribute to the good health of the baby as well as the mother. It contains disease-fighting antibodies to help protect babies from illness and it changes daily, weekly and monthly to meet their growing needs. Colostrum continues to protect the baby by giving them a special infection-fighting boost in the first few days after birth. Therefore breast fed babies have fewer infections and allergies and later in life are less likely to be obese.

If breast feeding is not possible, a formula milk should be used which should be made up according to the instructions. Non-cows' milk formula including soya-based infant formulas should only be used if a GP advises it. Babies who are allergic to cows' milk may also be allergic to soya.

Weaning and Onwards

Introducing solid foods, often called 'weaning', should start when a baby is around six months old. The latest research from the World Health Organisation shows that babies' digestive systems are not developed enough to cope with solid foods before they are around six months old. For bigger and more mature babies weaning should not occur before seventeen weeks of age. Giving a child a small mashed-up portion of whatever their carer is eating is not only cheap, but ensures that mothers know what has gone into their food, this is especially important if the family follows a special diet. A baby's diet should consist of a variety of the following types of food:

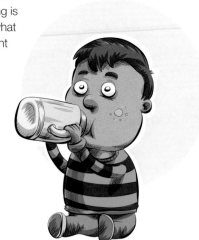

- Fruit and vegetables
- Bread, rice, pasta, potatoes and other starchy foods
- Meat, fish, eggs, beans and other non-dairy sources of protein
- Milk and dairy products.

Red meat (beef, pork and lamb) is an excellent source of protein. Eggs are also a quick and nutritious source of protein, but they must be cooked until both the white and yolk are solid. They are also a source of iron which infants can lack, as the store they are born with only lasts for 6 months. Extra salt and sugar should not be added to foods.

Whole cow's milk doesn't contain enough iron and other nutrients to meet babies' needs. It should not be given as a drink to babies under one year old, however, it is fine to use cows' milk when cooking and preparing food for a baby. Semi-skimmed milk can be introduced once a child is two years old, provided they are a good eater and have a varied diet. Skimmed milk is not suitable for children under five. For convenience, lower-fat milks can be used in cooking from the age of one.

By one year of age a child should be eating a balanced mixed diet. At the age of one year a child can be given full cream milk to drink instead of formula milk. At two years of age semi-skimmed milk can be introduced and at five years fully skimmed milk.

Children should be supervised when eating while they are learning to eat. Children can choke on nuts, sausages, grapes, boiled sweets and other round foods so these should be cut up.

Children and Teenagers

Children grow fast and should be very active. From the age of about five years they should be eating a diet in line with the eatwell plate. Teenagers grow quickly and about half of the calcium in the skeleton is deposited during the teenage years. Therefore plenty of calcium is needed. Girls start to menstruate during their teens, so a source of iron is required. Obesity and being overweight is increasingly a problem seen in children and teenagers, with up to 30% being overweight or obese.

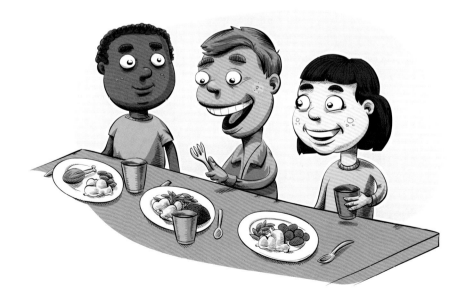

This extract from the British Heart Foundation Survey in 2008 shows a worrying trend in children's diets:

Nearly one in three UK kids (29%) is indulging by eating sweets, chocolate and crisps three or more times a day. And almost half of kids surveyed (40%) also admit they normally drink fizzy or energy drinks during the day. In contrast, almost nine in ten kids surveyed (88%) were not eating the recommended five portions of fruit and veg each day. In fact, children were more likely to have crisps at lunch (34%) than fruit (31%). With a third (32%) of children in England aged 11-15 now overweight or obese. A survey of 2,000 11 to 16 year olds helps give a unique snapshot of their daily diet. Based on the results, a child's typical daily diet includes one packet of crisps, one chocolate bar, one bag of chewy jelly sweets, one fizzy drink and one energy drink. That means kids are consuming almost 30 teaspoons of sugar (118g), more fat than a cheeseburger, and over a third of their daily calorie intake from snacks alone.

To improve the diet of young people there are standards in place regarding food in schools, which were produced by the Children's Food Trust. They include both food and nutrient standards.

Adults

According to government guidelines, adults should be eating a diet in line with the eatwell plate. Data published by the 'National Diet and Nutrition Survey', which looks at food consumption in the UK, shows that most adults should be eating more starchy foods. Starchy foods are a good source of energy and the main source of a range of nutrients in our diet. As well as starch, they contain fibre, calcium, iron and B vitamins.

- A maximum of 30-35% of total energy should come from fat
- A maximum of 10-11% of total energy should come from saturated fat
- A maximum of 2% of total energy should come from trans fat
- At least 45-50% total energy should come from carbohydrates
- A maximum of 10% of total energy should come from sugars
- A maximum of 15% of total energy should come from protein
- A maximum of 5% of total energy should come from alcohol (if used)

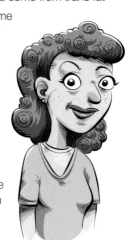
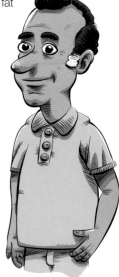

Deposits of fat around the waist and stomach, the so called 'apple shape', are particularly damaging to health and are linked with CHD, type 2 diabetes and high blood pressure. For this reason weight gain should be avoided.

Sport

For those engaged in sport, plenty of starchy carbohydrates are essential for energy. They also promote the development of glycogen, an energy store found in the liver and muscles, which assists with energy promotion.

Fluid is essential and due to perspiration, sports-people often need more than the usual two litres per day.

Pregnancy and Breast Feeding

A healthy diet is an important part of a healthy lifestyle at any time, but is vital during pregnancy or when planning a pregnancy. Eating healthily during pregnancy will help the baby to develop. Folic acid is recommended for the first twelve weeks of pregnancy to prevent neural tube defects.

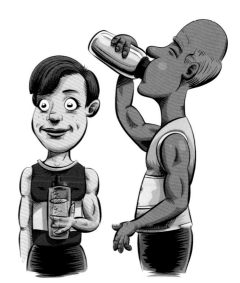

Eating plenty of fruit and vegetables is recommended because these provide vitamins and minerals, as well as fibre, which helps digestion and prevents constipation. The current advice is to eat at least five portions of fruit and vegetables a day. These can be fresh, frozen, canned, dried or juiced. Cook vegetables lightly in a little water, or eat them raw but well washed, to get the benefit of the nutrients they contain.

Starchy foods are an important source of vitamins and fibre, and are satisfying without containing too many calories. They include bread, potatoes, breakfast cereals, rice, pasta, noodles, maize, millet, oats, sweet potatoes, yams and cornmeal. These foods should be the main part of every meal. Eat wholemeal instead of processed (white) varieties for extra fibre.

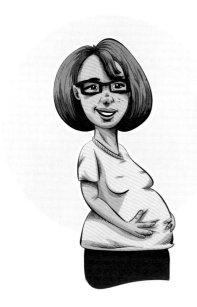

Sources of protein include meat, fish, poultry, eggs, beans, pulses and nuts. Those who are pregnant should eat some protein everyday but avoid liver due to its vitamin A content. Choose lean meat, remove the skin from poultry, and cook it using only a little fat. Make sure eggs, poultry, pork, burgers and sausages are cooked all the way through. Check that there is no pink meat, and that juices have no pink or red in them. Two portions of fish a week are recommended, one of which should be oily fish such as sardines or mackerel. There are some types of fish to avoid in pregnancy such as shark and marlin, due to their mercury content.

Dairy foods such as milk, cheese, fromage frais and yoghurt are important because they contain calcium and other nutrients that are needed. Choose low-fat varieties wherever possible, such as semi-skimmed or skimmed milk, low-fat yoghurt and half-fat hard cheese. Aim for two to three portions a day. There are some cheeses to avoid such as unpasteurised brie and camembert.

Sugar contains calories without providing any other nutrients, and can contribute to weight gain, obesity and tooth decay. Fat is very high in calories, and eating more fatty foods is likely to make pregnant women gain excesss weight.

For breast feeding, a well balanced diet in line with the eatwell plate is recommended, with extra fluid, particularly milk for the extra calcium it provides. Most mothers who breastfeed are advised to take supplements of vitamin D.

Older People

A healthy diet in line with the eatwell plate encourages healthy ageing. Older people need to ensure they are getting enough calcium, iron, vitamin D, fluid and fibre.

Some older people have problems with the foods they eat due to dental problems, difficulty in cooking and difficulties in obtaining shopping. Some elderly people may be malnourished and careful planning of food intake to ensure extra calories are consumed may be required.

The Care Quality Commission (CQC) is responsible for checking that residential homes and hospitals meet national standards. They have regulations on meeting nutritional needs which includes an emphasis on food and hydration.

There should be:

- A choice of suitable food and hydration in sufficient quantities to meet the service users' needs
- Food and hydration to meet any reasonable requirements from service users' religious or cultural background
- Support where needed for the purpose of enabling service users to eat and drink sufficient amounts.

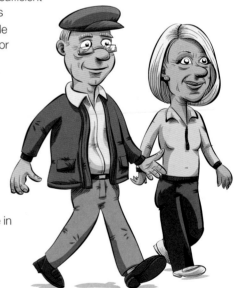

Various initiatives have been involved in promoting good nutrition in older people, including support in the community by means of delivered meals and lunch clubs.

Those who are malnourished or ill will require tempting high calorie foods which may not be in line with the eatwell plate.

Reader Reflection

Plan a diet for a young pregnant women who is a vegetarian and how you would ensure she has a balanced diet.

Good Catering Practices

Information Sources

Registered Dietitians (RDs) are the only qualified health professionals who assess, diagnose and treat diet and nutrition problems at an individual and wider public health level. Uniquely, dietitians use the most up to date public health and scientific research on food, health and disease, which they translate into practical guidance to enable people to make appropriate lifestyle and food choices. Dietitians are the only nutrition professionals to be statutorily regulated, and governed by an ethical code, to ensure that they always work to the highest standard. Dietitians work in the NHS, private practice, industry, education, research, sport, media, public relations, publishing, NGOs and government. Their advice influences food and health policy across the spectrum from government, local communities and individuals. The title Dietitian can only be used by those appropriately trained professionals who have registered with the Health Professions Council.

Food Packs

Food packs are useful sources of information about foods and the nutrients they contain. By law, food packs must show a list of ingredients. The ingredients are listed in order of weight in descending order, ending with those in the smallest quantity and this is often a list of additives. Manufacturers can put either the full name of the additive or its E number. An E number means that a food additive is permitted to be used throughout the EU. Packs must also provide information on the product name, the manufacturer's name, the weight of the pack and any special storage instructions. Allergens must also be shown.

Dates are required information on food labels: a use by date for perishable items like chilled meals or cooked meats and best before dates on non-perishable items like flour, canned items or crisps. Perishable items are a food safety risk if eaten after the use by date. It is also an offence to sell them after the use by date. Food eaten after the best before date may not taste as good, for example crisps may go soggy.

Manufacturers can only make a claim about the nutrient content of a food and not about any health benefits. For example, they can say a food is low in fat but not that it prevents illnesses. If they make claims about the health benefits of a food, it must be backed up by extensive research.

Nutritional information does not need to be put on foods but most manufacturers do place it on labels. If a claim is put on a label such as low fat or high fibre, then nutritional information must be provided. This must be given per 100g or per 100ml. The following is put on food labels:

- Energy kJ
- Energy kcal
- Carbohydrate
- Sugars
- Fat
- Saturates
- Protein
- Fibre
- Sodium (salt equivalents)

Food manufacturers use both traffic light colour coding and percentage Guideline Daily Amounts (GDAs) on food labels. The percentage GDA shows what percentage of calories, fat, saturated fat, carbohydrate, sugars, protein, fibre and salt a food contains.

NUTRITION INFORMATION			GUIDELINE DAILY AMOUNTS		
Typical values	per 100g	per 350g serving	Women	Men	Children (5-10 years)
Energy – kj	480kj	1680kj			
– kcal (Calories)	115kcal	405kcal	2000	2500	1800
Protein	9.5g	33.3g	45g	55g	24g
Carbohydrate	8.6g	30.1g	230g	300g	220g
of which sugars	2.0g	7.0g	90g	120g	85g
Fat	4.6g	16.1g	70g	95g	70g
of which saturates	3.0g	10.0g	20g	30g	20g
Fibre	1.5g	5.3g	24g	24g	15g
Sodium*	0.3g	1.1g	2.4g	2.4g	1.4g
*Equivalent as salt	0.8g	2.8g	6g	6g	4g

Manufacturers may also use a traffic light system. Traffic lights indicate whether a food is high (red), medium (amber) or low (green) in sugar, total fat, saturated fat and salt.

On food labels the following figures are used according to the red, amber or green light system.

- A high amount of sugar is more than 15g per 100g and
- A low amount of sugar is 5g per 100g

- A high amount of fat is more than 20g per 100g and
- A low amount of fat is 3g per 100g

- A high amount of saturated fat is more than 5g per 100g and
- A low amount of saturated fat is 1.5g per 100g

- A high amount of salt is more than 1.5g per 100g (0.6g sodium) and
- A low amount of salt is 0.3g per 100g (0.1g sodium).

Healthier Catering Practices

In schools and care homes fluid should be available to drink at all times. This is also good practice in other work situations.

In menus, five portions of fruit and vegetables (80g per portion) should be available each day. Fruit juice can form one of the portions, but as it contains little fibre it cannot count as more than one portion per day no matter how much is provided. A variety of fruit and vegetables can provide a wide range of vitamins as well as antioxidants.

To retain the vitamins in fruit and vegetables try to eat them fresh and, if possible, do not peel them. Steam rather than boil them or cook by microwaving or boiling in a small amount of water. Cook quickly and do not keep them warm for long periods. Use any cooking water in soups or sauces. Do not add bicarbonate of soda as this destroys vitamin C. Frozen vegetables retain their vitamins. Canned fruits and vegetables have less vitamin C than fresh alternatives, but still provide some and are useful store cupboard standbys. Choosing fruit canned in juice or vegetables with reduced salt, is a healthier option.

Increase Fibre

Fibre can be increased in diets by various simple techniques such as:

- Using a small amount of wholemeal flour alongside white flour in baking
- Using wholemeal bread or a white high-fibre bread
- Using brown pasta and brown rice in dishes.
- Adding fruit and vegetables to various dishes. For example, make home made soups with vegetables or add extra vegetables to dishes such as lasagne and shepherds pie. Vegetables can also be used in cakes such as carrot cake and chocolate beetroot cake. Fruit puddings can be used often, such as crumbles and pies with a deep filling of fruit.

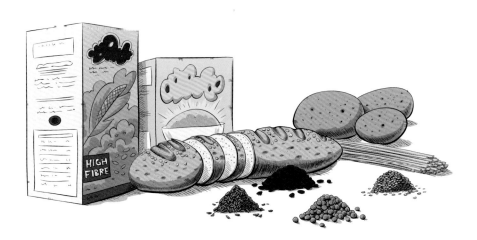

Reduce Saturated Fat

- Avoid frying in lard and use a polyunsaturated margarine instead
- Use rapeseed oil for frying
- Use less pastry by only having a thin topping on pies
- Use semi/skimmed milk in custard and desserts

Reduce Sugar

- Avoid adding sugar to cereals and drinks, cut down gradually so that less is needed
- Use dried fruit for sweetening in cakes, pastries and puddings
- Use less sugar in items such as soft drinks and jams
- Use less sugar in baking than the recipe suggests
- Choose fruit canned in juice

Reduce Salt

- Avoid adding salt when cooking
- Use herbs and spices for added flavour
- Use more fresh vegetables than canned ones
- Avoid using ready made dishes

Increase Calories

This is important for those who are malnourished and can be achieved if you:

- Use more butter, cheese and fats in dishes such as in mashed potatoes
- Use cream in porridge and puddings
- Use full cream milk in cooking
- Tempt with sugary items such as cakes and desserts

Promotion

Promoting a healthy diet is important both to tempt and encourage people to eat healthily. This can be achieved with:

- Posters of various pieces of information including the eatwell plate
- Information about dishes as well as recipes
- Tasting sessions of healthier dishes particularly those with extra fruit and vegetables
- Leaflets about health and diet
- Meal deals of healthier foods
- Cookery demonstrations that include ways of making food look appealing

Reader Reflection

Suggest ways you could promote a healthier diet to your family and also in your workplace.

Summary

The information on various aspects of food and nutrition that you have studied should have informed and inspired you to put into practice what you have learnt. This will be of benefit both to you and those you cater or care for.

Future

It is hoped this will have inspired you to go on to do further studies in the area of food and health and the following RSPH qualifications may be of interest.

There is also a comprehensive list of resources at the end of this book to provide you with more information.

1. **Level 2 Award in Healthier Food and Special Diets**
This qualification is aimed at those involved in catering, food and health-related occupations, and also to carers, community workers, fitness trainers and other individuals who have a role in the promotion of health. It would also be appropriate as part of lifestyle education for people of all ages, and especially for young people.

2. **Level 3 Award in Nutrition for Healthier Food and Special Diets**
This qualification is suitable for people working in catering and others who are in a position to promote healthy nutrition. It is relevant for employees of health-related companies, and for people working in the health, caring or teaching professions who might have a role in the promotion of healthy eating or the preparation of meals, menus and diets.

3. **Level 3 Certificate in Nutrition and Health**
This examination is designed for anyone interested in the practical application of the principles of nutrition and healthy eating. The Certificate is a particularly useful qualification for those working in the following areas: hotel and catering industries; caring professions; retail food trades; health and beauty industries and food manufacturing.

4. **Level 4 Award in Nutrition**
This qualification is designed for anyone interested in the practical application of the principles of nutrition and healthy eating. This Award is particularly suited to anyone working in hotel and catering industries; caring professions; retail food trades; health and beauty industries and food manufacturing industries.

5. **Level 4 Certificate in Nutrition**
This qualification is designed for more specialist study of the application of the principles of nutrition and healthy eating. There are two options available for anyone who wishes to focus either on sport's nutrition or on catering for particular service sectors.

Reader Reflection

Think of two key things that you have learnt and that you can apply in practice.

Resources

Useful NHS and Department of Health information www.nhs.uk/LiveWell

Useful NHS and Department of Health information – Change 4 life deals with health and diet through all life stages www.nhs.uk/change4life/pages/cut-back-on-fat.aspx

The Food Standards Agency site, which has information on food safety www.food.gov.uk

The Food Standards Agency site, which has information on food allergy http://allergytraining.food.gov.uk

The Children's Food Trust has information on all aspects of food in schools www.childrensfoodtrust.org.uk

Information on dental health and diet www.dentalhealth.org

Information on all aspects of alcohol and health www.drinkaware.co.uk

Information on diabetes www.diabetes.org.uk

Information on diabetes www.iddt.org

Information on nutritional assessment using the MUST tool www.bapen.org.uk

Information on vegan diets www.vegansociety.

Information on vegetarian diets www.vegsoc.org

Information on gluten free diets www.coeliac.org.uk

Information on diet and health and the role of registered dietitians www.bda.uk.com

Information on nutrition and older people www.ageuk.org.uk

Information on food available in supermarkets as well as calorie content of foods www.mysupermarket.co.uk

Books

McCance and Widdowson's the Composition of Foods: Summary Edition, Royal Society of Chemistry; 6th Revised edition (1 Sep 2002) ISBN-10: 0854044280 ISBN-13: 978-0854044283.

Manual of Nutrition by Food Standards Stationery Office; 11th ed., 2008 edition (9 May 2008) Language: English ISBN-10: 011243116X ISBN-13: 978-0112431169.